HYPOTHYROIDISM DIAGNOSIS GUIDE

Signs, Systems, Treatments, and Vital Information To Help You Live with Hypothyroidism

Kathryn Young

SPECIAL BONUS

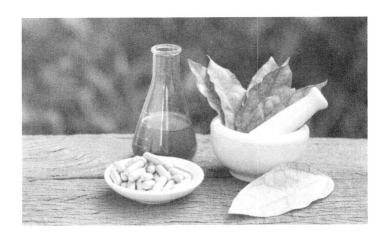

Get the Bonus Report that includes:

❏ Weight loss supplement buying guide
❏ Why **MOST** diets fail
❏ Alternative medicine tricks that worked for
me

Get it now, visit the link:

bit.ly/healthybonus

TABLE OF CONTENTS

INTRODUCTION

"The question isn't how to get cured but how to live."

- Joseph Courad,

Hypothyroidism has appeared in many search histories lately, most likely yours included.

Whether you are looking for answers due to unexplained symptoms or have received a diagnosis of your own, your health is important. Understanding the long-term implications of this condition will better direct you to a healthier tomorrow.

One of the most credible fears is fear of the unknown. Living a life, without knowing and understanding your situation or condition, you may become fearful of what you don't know.

For example:

If someone is experiencing chest pains, their fear may be much worse than the real issue. Chest pains could be gas or a heart attack, either way you should find out.

Your thyroid is as crucial as your cardiac health. Your thyroid gland controls many aspects of your body's functions. Because so many of your body's systems depend upon it, your thyroid is a crucial part of your health.

In this book you will gain insight into the condition, its symptoms (even the ancient ones), and how they impact you. You will also learn the steps available to you to seek medical attention to be on the way to a healthier you. We will also look at the benefits of early diagnosis, and the varying styles you can choose control right away.

As with any health diagnosis, the earlier, the better. With cancer, catching it early on allows for more treatment options, a higher probability of being able to stop the disease before it spreads, and a better treatment plan. If you wait too long, your condition could become worse, and treatment becomes harder and success rates go down. You are putting yourself in a much better position by seeking medical attention as soon as possible.

If something feels wrong, start looking into it as soon as possible. In this case, you or someone that you are close to has most likely already picked up on and acknowledged symptoms that are not common in your daily life. You may need some time for a professional to pinpoint the problem, which will lead to a solution. Only then can you determine if hypothyroidism is the leading cause.

According to the American Thyroid Association, more than 12 percent of the population within the United States will have some condition with their thyroid. This means that right around 20 million individuals are living with some form of thyroid disease. And about 60 percent of those who have thyroid disease, have no idea that they have a condition. Left untreated, hypothyroidism can create and lead to countless other issues and ailments that, with proper attention could be nonissues.

You are already one step ahead!

Hypothyroidism will no longer hold you back in all aspects of your life as it does now. It's not about finding a quick fix or a cure with medication. This is about finding the correct balance of changes, medical collaboration, and becoming informed and educated on what is going on with your body.

Whether you're new to gathering information on thyroid disease or are a seasoned patient living with hypothyroidism, you will find information to carry you to new perspectives on the condition to figure out how to make thyroid disease work for you.

You've completed the first step by taking action and seeking out information.

From here, let's get you informed. The time is now!

CHAPTER 1

START WITH THE BASICS: WHAT IS HYPOTHYROIDISM?

"I've gained weight."

"I'm sleepy all the time. All I want to do is sleep."

"My hair is thinning."

"Can you pick up some fiber from the store? I'm constipated."

"I need a facial and my skin is dry."

"I'm weak."

While many of these statements sound much like stress and old age, they're also symptoms of hypothyroidism.

When you are under a lot of pressure, you wake up, and you are already tired. You can gain weight from stress. Yet, these are also some of the symptoms of hypothyroidism.

These symptoms are prevalent among other symptoms and conditions presented by many other conditions, it can be challenging to identify whether their symptoms are being brought on by hypothyroidism.

What is Hypothyroidism, Anyways?

Your thyroid is a gland that is positioned at the front of your neck, below your larynx, or Adam's Apple, shaped like a butterfly. You can actually feel your thyroid, and when you apply pressure to that area of your neck.

The thyroid gland handles releasing hormones that regulate your metabolic rate, which, in turn, maintains and adjusts your digestive, heart, and muscle function. Your thyroid gland also plays a part in bone maintenance and brain development.

Your thyroid dictates how the cells of your body use the energy they absorb from food. This is your metabolism, which has a direct effect on your body's temperature, your heartbeat, and even how efficient your body is at burning calories.

When your body lacks thyroid hormone, your normal body functions, and processes slow down. As this happens, your metabolism takes a hit and slows down, and that's why you have less energy.

Lacking thyroid hormone is known as hypothyroidism. Hypothyroidism is a condition in which your body is not producing a large number of thyroid hormones.

Some refer to hypothyroidism as "underactive thyroid."

What's the difference between hypothyroidism and hyperthyroidism?

For those with hypothyroidism, the thyroid does not produce a large amount of thyroid hormone for your body to function.

The main difference between hypothyroidism versus hyperthyroidism is the quantity of hormones produced.

To keep in simple:
Hypo - not enough thyroid hormones
Hyper - excess of thyroid hormones

Because hyperthyroidism produces more thyroid hormones, this causes your metabolism to speed up. On the flip side, if you are diagnosed with hypothyroidism, your metabolism will slow down.

With both hypothyroidism and hyperthyroidism, you are always on either side of the spectrum. They are polar opposites. If you have hypothyroidism, you are likely to be cold, and if you have hyperthyroidism, you may not tolerate heat too well. This means that in a perfect world with a functioning thyroid, you should be in the middle in a happy medium.

That's why treatments for hypothyroidism and hyperthyroidism act to get you in a happy medium.

Who Does Hypothyroidism Affect?

It should be noted that hypothyroidism affects women more often than men. Hypothyroidism is common in people over the age of 60, but one can begin to develop the condition at any age.

An expert and associate professor of medicine and endocrinology at Georgetown University School of Medicine in Washington, D.C., weighed in on the subject:

"We do not understand the reason for women being more susceptible to developing hypothyroidism, but it is at least in part because Hashimoto's hypothyroidism — the most common cause of hypothyroidism in the United States — is an autoimmune disease," said Jacqueline Jonklaas, MD, Ph.D., MPH,

"Autoimmune diseases are, in general, more common in women."

There are some symptoms that are gender specific as they relate to the reproductive systems. Infertility, although much more common in women than in men, can come from hypothyroidism. Galactorrhea, a discharge from a woman's breasts, is rare but is also something that only women can experience as a result of hypothyroidism.

Because females struggle more with issues with their thyroid gland, men are sometimes overlooked. For both males and females, libido is seldom affected, and men can struggle with erectile dysfunction.

Far too often, medical professionals can overlook problems with a low thyroid level, ignoring the signals and symptoms and failing to piece together because men are sometimes forgotten when it comes to thyroid problems. Male patients sometimes overlook the signs more than females and wonder if they imagine things, while doctors imply that they're stressed out or getting older.

Men can experience balding, and many of the symptom's females endure, but they have their own concerns and problems. While women usually have

9

unexplained and quick weight gain, men are on the opposite end. They may actually lose muscle mass and some of their strength.

Unknown to most, a low thyroid can have a vast increase in the number of sperm cells of the testicles with a much lower count of mature sperm cells. In male patients, this larger testicular size goes hand in hand with poor sperm quality. It is said that there may be a direct correlation between hypothyroidism and sperm count.

Hypothyroidism and Babies

Babies can have hypothyroidism. In infants, it's known as congenital hypothyroidism (CH). Symptoms for babies are a little different than the norm. When treated right away upon that early diagnosis, the babies will usually grow out of it by the age of three. They are believed to have a transient or short-term version of the condition.

The most common reason for a baby to have congenital hypothyroidism is the thyroid gland failing to completely develop before birth. Sometimes, the pancreas appears to be present, but it cannot produce the thyroid hormones necessary for normal functioning. On other occasions, the thyroid gland is formed in an area in the infant's neck that is not normal.

This provides for abnormal or malfunctioning thyroid glands. The condition is sometimes also brought on if the mother is treated for a thyroid condition while pregnant with that baby. The mother's diet can also impact that baby during pregnancy. If her food is deficient in iodine, her child can also suffer from low thyroid hormone levels when the baby is born.

Some, if not most babies, have no clear signs of hypothyroidism at birth. The condition is only picked up on by a blood test. Yet, sometimes, some symptoms that babies may encounter are a hoarse cry, a puffy face, a thick tongue, lethargy, or even a distended stomach. Some other possible symptoms that may come with congenital hypothyroidism in little babies are constipation, feeding problems, slow bone growth, and a large fontanelle (a soft spot on the top of a baby's head), dry skin, and weak muscles. As with adults, many of these symptoms can apply to other conditions, and coupled with the fact that many new parents are very new to babies and their health, linking them with hypothyroidism can be difficult.

Hypothyroidism in Children and Teenagers

When hypothyroidism is present in children and teenagers, for the most part, they display the same symptoms that adults do. But there are some signs and symptoms that only children encounter. Kids can show signs of weak growth, usually ending in short stature. Some symptoms are a delayed development of their permanent teeth and they can undergo late onset of puberty and even poor mental development.

What Causes Hypothyroidism?

Your immune system provides one primary function to your body: to protect your organization's cells against harmful bacteria, germs, and viruses. When foreign bacteria or viruses enter into your body through your eyes, nose, and mouth, your immune system jumps into action and responds by releasing "fighter cells" to battle and take down the foreign cells. These fighter cells are actually a type of protein called antibodies, and they fight off common ailments and illnesses such as the flu or a common cold. They assist in protecting you against severe illnesses such as cancer or even heart disease.

Sometimes, your body confuses your primary and healthy cells in your body for the foreign invading cells. This is also known as an *autoimmune response*. Your immune system may go after healthy tissues within your body if this autoimmune response is not taken cared of or regulated. This is what then leads to possible medical problems such as hypothyroidism.

Hashimoto's disease is a type of hypothyroidism and is actually an autoimmune condition brought on by an under-active thyroid. This condition actually attacks your thyroid gland and can lead to thyroid inflammation, leading to poor thyroid function. It is very common that many members of the same family have this condition.

Some medicines will get in the way of your thyroid's ability to produce the thyroid hormone. This, by itself, can lead to hypothyroidism. Some other types of drugs that can cause hypothyroidism are interferon-alpha, amiodarone, lithium, and interleukin-2.

All these medications will likely trigger hypothyroidism in individuals with a genetic specific tendency to autoimmune thyroid disease.

While it's sporadic, some individuals who struggle with many myelomas are at risk of developing hypothyroidism.

Your body's pituitary gland tells your thyroid gland the correct amount of hormone to produce. If the pituitary gland ends up being damaged by injury, surgery, tumors, or even corrective radiation, communication to the thyroid may be broken. It may not be able to instruct the thyroid gland. Thus, your thyroid may not make enough thyroid hormones any longer.

Hashimoto's Disease

The most common cause of hypothyroidism is Hashimoto's Disease, an autoimmune disorder. An autoimmune disorder is any condition that occurs and then your immune system begins to attack your body. It is unknown what causes your immune system to go after your own body, but, after some research, it is said that women are much more prone to the many types of autoimmune disorder than men are. In fact, women get these types of diseases at a 2 to 1 ratio to men. Some other examples of autoimmune disorders are lupus and sclerosis, and some of these conditions are more prevalent in specific ethnic groups, or they run in particular families.

Autoimmune disorders happen when your immune system yields specific antibodies that wind up going after your own body's tissues. Sometimes, this will include your thyroid gland, which, in turn, affects your thyroid's ability to produce hormones, if at all.

Many times, a woman will develop Hashimoto's after having a baby. Sometimes, the condition will go away shortly after.

It must be noted that hypothyroidism and Hashimoto's Disease are *two separate things*, not interchangeable terms for the same condition. It is possible to suffer from Hashimoto's without being hypothyroid. Yet, most people with Hashimoto's Disease do develop hypothyroidism over time. Remember that hypothyroidism has to do with your thyroid gland and Hashimoto's has to do with your immune system.

While they work together at times, these are separate conditions.

Birth Control and Hypothyroidism

It should be noted that your thyroid hormones work side by side with your sex hormones. Estrogen, progesterone, and testosterone all have an impact on each other. When you are ingesting sex hormones via birth control pills, the estrogen and progesterone that make up the tiny pills you take can impact your body's thyroid-binding proteins, which will increase the amount. This means that if you have hypothyroidism, all your medications' dosages must be increased while you're on oral contraceptives to counteract the extra sex hormones. This also means that when you stop taking the pills, your prescription will need to be lowered.

It is said that any oral contraceptive that contains the hormone progesterone has the potential to increase your body's T3 and T4 levels.

Birth Control and Hashimoto's Disease

Sex hormones are also known to impact the immune system, thus affecting Hashimoto's.

Varying types of oral hormonal contraception and even some types of hormone therapy are known to impact your thyroid in many ways. We know that taking birth control pills can affect your thyroid hormone levels. Taking a more in-depth look, we see that Combined Oral Contraceptives, also known as COCs, are a form of birth control.

COCs have ethinyl estradiol, a type of estrogen, and progestin, a variety of progesterone. It has been proven that taking COCs affects adrenal function as well as your thyroid.

Looking Deeper at the Symptoms
Fatigue

There is a massive connection between fatigue and hypothyroidism. Experiencing fatigue and being tired all the time is one of the telltale signs of hypothyroidism. Many individuals diagnosed with the condition say that they are always so sleepy that they are unable to have a typical day and get things done because they are tired. The fatigue will take hold, regardless of how much that person sleeps and for how long.

This fatigue can come on a little bit at a time, or all at once, leaving you over-exhausted and cranky.

Treating the condition is found to improve the energy levels of those with hypothyroidism.

Sore Muscles and Joints

Your muscles and joints can also become affected, and you may experience aches, pains, weakness, stiffness, tenderness, and even swelling. A link has also been found between thyroid issues and rheumatoid arthritis, plagued by excruciating swelling in your joints.

Mood Changes

Hypothyroidism may bring on a lot of mood-related problems. These can include depression, low moods, slower cognitive skills and speech, anxiety, apathy, feelings of indifference, and lapses in memory. These all occur because your brain relies on thyroid hormones to operate and function and at its full potential. Upon treatment, these symptoms, while scary, are reversible.

Depression is a massive issue in those with hypothyroidism. More than half of those with hypothyroidism report feelings of depression.

Weight Gain

Fluctuations in your weight happen, based on diet and exercise. But unexplained gains in your body are the problem here. Everyone's thyroid hormones aid in regulating one's body weight, intake of food, and the metabolic process your body undergoes when consuming food—It metabolites fat and sugar.

You may have unexplained weight gain and experience an increase in your body mass index (BMI).

Even if you have a mild hypothyroidism case, you may experience weight gain and even obesity down the road. Those who struggle with hypothyroidism will often document that they notice a puffier face and extra weight around their stomach or other body areas as a symptom.

Feeling Cold All the Time (Or Most of the Time)

Hypothyroidism, as we know, slows down your metabolism. This has the potential to lead to a decrease in your core body temperature. As a result, you may feel chilly all or most of the time. You will also most likely experience a low tolerance for any cold conditions.

Even on the beach, or in a warm or even hot area, you may still feel cold. Those struggling with hypothyroidism often have cold hands and feet, even if they don't think it's hot anywhere else.

Slow Heart Rate

Hypothyroidism may also lead you to have a slower than usual heart rate. This is also known as bradycardia. Hypothyroidism doesn't affect only your heart rate, but it can impact your blood pressure, heart rhythm, and arteries.

It should be noted that bradycardia can lead to a sense of weakness, dizziness, or breathing issues. This now brings on a whole range of other items to be concerned with as well.

Your heart is essential, and without treatment, any cardiac issue or condition could lead to severe complications, such as both high and/or low blood pressure or even heart failure.

Hair Loss

Like other hormone disorders, hypothyroidism can contribute and lead to hair loss. We're talking in large clumps in some cases! This occurs because thyroid hormones are essential to support the health and growth of hair follicles. You could lose your hair from the scalp, arms, legs, eyebrows, and pretty much anywhere that hair grows on your body.

High Cholesterol

Your thyroid hormones play an essential role in the ridding of excess cholesterol from your body through your liver. Low thyroid hormone levels lead to your liver struggling to free the leftover cholesterol. As a result, your blood cholesterol levels are at risk of increasing and amount to dangerous levels.

There's a connection between hypothyroidism and high cholesterol, It's said that up to 13 percent of those with higher than normal cholesterol levels also struggle with hypothyroidism. Because of this, many experts recommend that all doctors check for thyroid problems in those with high cholesterol levels.

In turn, treating and correcting your thyroid issue

may actually help to get your cholesterol levels back on track, even without any particular medication.

Constipation

Constipation: not fun! While we are talking about thyroids that are too slow, let's talk about how hypothyroidism also slows down your digestion. Studies have proven that when your thyroid is too slow and sluggish, it can lead to issues with food movement through your gut, and it slows down your stomach, colon, and small intestine. These digestive issues can lead to constipation.

By constipation, we mean less than three bowel movements in a week.

Always be ready with some laxatives!

You may also have hard and firm stools, problems going #2, or a feeling that you are never done going to the bathroom.

Skin, Hair, and Nails

Issues and problems with your thyroid can also affect your skin in many different ways and can lead to symptoms such as dry, thin, or scaly skin and paleness. Your hair may become very dried out or brittle, and your nails may become dull and weak, breakable.

Menstrual Changes

Females with hypothyroidism may go through very heavy or even irregular menstrual periods. Spotting between these periods may also occur. This happens because hypothyroidism diminishes the amount of sex hormone-binding, globulin.

The condition also creates issues with how the body detoxifies estrogen.

Anemia

Anemia is the most prevalent blood disorder of all. It's characterized by a low count on the number of red blood cells circulating in your circulatory system. It can sometimes be the first sign of hypothyroidism.

This can lead to feeling tired, dizzy, shortness of breath, and heart-pounding. When your red blood cell count is low, this can lead to an array of other issues.

Sleep Apnea

There is a link between hypothyroidism and sleep apnea. Sleep apnea is when some brief times while you are sleeping that you stop breathing. Those that suffer from sleep apnea are big snorers also. When you stop breathing from time to time, the amount of oxygen that your body receives becomes limited, and this leads to sleep disruption and brings on even more exhaustion. Sleep apnea can then lead to diabetes, low blood oxygen levels, abnormal cholesterol, heart disease, memory loss, mental confusion, depression, and a weakened immune system.

Goiter

A goiter can appear in your neck if you have hypothyroidism. When your thyroid gland becomes enlarged, there's swelling at the base of your neck, and this goiter occurs. The goiter can be uncomfortable and may lead to your voice being hoarse, a persistent cough, and difficulties breathing and swallowing.

Disclaimer

If you are struggling with hypothyroidism, you may be experiencing some other body changes that you cannot pick up on or even feel. It can be tough to know that excessive amounts of cholesterol are building up in your body's blood or that plaque is thickening in your arteries' walls. These are things that can lead to cardiac issues. Hypothyroidism brings about pesky and annoying symptoms, but it can also worsen other health issues, making for severe problems.

The most challenging problem, with the symptoms that hypothyroidism brings on is that they are very like the things that happen to your body as your natural age.

This is why hypothyroidism is often missed.

https://www.thyroid.org/media-main/press-room/

https://www.yourhormones.info/glands/thyroid-gland/

https://health.usnews.com/health-news/patient-advice/articles/2015/07/21/low-thyroid-in-men-not-just-a-womans-issue https://www.healthline.com/health/autoimmune-disorders#causes

]https://www.endocrineweb.com/conditions/thyroid/low-thyroid-level-newborns-new-clues-how-treat

https://www.health.harvard.edu/diseases-and-conditions/the-lowdown-on-thyroid-slowdown

CHAPTER 2

THE JOURNEY TO HYPOTHYROIDISM DIAGNOSIS

People don't always showcase the same symptoms. Some may display all, some may struggle with a combination of them, and some may have very slight variations of the symptoms outlined before. Usually, people do not reach a diagnosis unless they first have a reason to look into their medical condition.

It's more uncommon for hypothyroidism to be seen on a blood lab report than to diagnose by sorting through symptoms and then beginning to conduct tests, labs, and bloodwork.

Because we're all different, and nobody can predict which symptoms an individual may develop or how severe the symptoms may end up being, the only way to be sure if you have hypothyroidism is through blood tests.

For some individuals, the process can take some time.

The journey to a diagnosis begins once you begin to look into your symptoms and seek medical help. You may encounter a lengthy and stressful period of trial and error while trying to identify hypothyroidism because your symptoms can be mistaken with other conditions.

If you are displaying the symptoms, confirm with your doctor to test if you have hypothyroidism.

Testing for Hypothyroidism

When your thyroxine levels are low, and your TSH levels are high, this can indicate that you may have hypothyroidism. This happens as a result of your pituitary gland as it will create more TSH in an attempt to help your thyroid gland to generate more thyroid hormone.

Doctors can diagnose thyroid disorders sooner than ever before. It's believed that testing your TSH levels is the best way to check for hypothyroidism. As a result, your doctor may check your TSH levels first and then follow up with a T4 test if necessary.

TSH tests are the primary way to maintain and figure out the best dosage of medication to start with and then to find the perfect dosage.

Testing your TSH levels is also very important to try to diagnose a sickness known as subclinical hypothyroidism. This condition does'nt have any signs or symptoms. If you have subclinical hypothyroidism, you will have regular blood levels of triiodothyronine and thyroxine. You'll also have some higher than usual levels of TSH.

What Can Affect Your Bloodwork?

There are a few factors that can come into play and affect your blood tests for hypothyroidism.

Heparin, a blood thinner, can have an impact on the results of your bloodwork. Another is a vitamin supplement known as biotin which can also skew your results. It's important to let your doctor know exactly which medications and supplements you've taken days before the blood test to get the most accurate results back.

TSH Levels

According to the American Thyroid Association, these are normal TSH Levels:

NORMAL AND ABNORMAL TSH LEVELS (mU/L)

TSH LEVELS MEASURED THROUGH BLOOD TESTS:

TSH AND T4 BLOOD TESTS
0.0 – 0.4

Hyperthyroidism or Suppressed TSH
0.4 – 4.0

The Normal Range of TSH
4.0 - 10.0 10.00 +

Subclinical (mild) Hypothyroidism
In most labs, the normal range for TSH
0.4 mU/L to 4.0 mU/L

If your TSH levels come back at above 4.0 mU/L, you may have hypothyroidism.

Most people with a functioning thyroid gland have levels of TSH that are between
0.4 mU/L and 4.0 mU/L.

T4

T4 is made and synthesized by your thyroid gland. The "free T4" and the "free T4 index" are fancy ways of talking about the blood tests combined with your TSH test to give a mixed result.

When your results from TSH and T4 are analyzed together, a doctor can better check your thyroid function.

In most cases, if the findings are that you have a lower than usual level of T4 coupled with a higher than average TSH level, you most likely have hypothyroidism.

Analyzing Your Thyroid Levels

By looking at your thyroid blood levels, your doctor will be looking for a few things.

If your TSH levels fall somewhere between 0.45 and 4.5 mU/L, you don't have hypothyroidism and are healthy. If your TSH is high and somewhere above 4.5 mU/L and your free T4 is standard, somewhere between 0.8–2.0 ng/dL, you may have subclinical hypothyroidism.

It should be noted that there isn't a standard way to treat subclinical hypothyroidism. Most doctors usually plan their course of treatment based on the symptoms you present and your family history. This may involve a bunch of trial and error with treatments and medications to find something that works for you.

If your TSH levels are high and your T4 low, you most likely are dealing with an under-active thyroid, and treatment is necessary.

What will your doctor need to know?

When you're with your doctor, he or she will most likely inquire about your symptoms.

Your doctor will want to know when the symptoms started, the severity of your symptoms, if your symptoms come and go, or if they are continuous and if anything helps to reduce your symptoms. They will also ask if you've noticed if anything makes these symptoms worse.

So it's incredibly important to pay attention to your symptoms.

Medical History

You must tell your doctor everything you can disclose. Your personal medical history is essential to discuss, as well as your family's history.

A doctor may inquire about changes in your health to see if you or anyone in your family were ever diagnosed with any thyroid problem. If you've had thyroid surgery and radiation on your neck, and if you are taking any of the medications that were earlier discussed, it may cause hypothyroidism.

How Can Hypothyroidism NOT be diagnosed?

It's important to discuss and note the ways that hypothyroidism can't be detected.

You should not base it on 3 things:

- Body temperature will not work because a healthy individual and someone who has hypothyroidism can both have average temperatures of 98.6 degrees Fahrenheit.
- Slow reflexes and saliva tests are also not good indicators as they aren't deemed to be accurate.
- Going off of your neck size is not active. Hypothyroidism does not show any change in

their neck size and never develops a goiter.

For more information, check these links below:

https://www.thyroid.org/wp-content/uploads/patients/brochures/Hypothyroidism_web_booklet.pdf

https://www.health.harvard.edu/diseases-and-conditions/the-lowdown-on-thyroid-slowdown

CHAPTER 3

HYPOTHYROIDISM TREATMENTS: NO ONE-SIZE-FITS-ALL APPROACH

There is usually one mainstream medication type that is relied on to treat hypothyroidism. It's said that hypothyroidism is best handled by prescribing the medication known as levothyroxine.

It's a synthetic version of your T4 hormones (levothyroxine sodium), and it takes on and mimics what your thyroid hormone would do inside your body.

Levothyroxine can be purchased in the generic form and under some other brands such as Synthroid, Levothroid, and Levoxyl.

These medications will contain the exact same synthetic T4, but their inactive ingredients can be different. This isn't usually an issue, but for some people, the idle ingredient variations may affect the absorption of the synthetic T4.

As a result, once you are on a particular brand and working for you, you should not switch it up. If your pharmacy ever switches to a generic version, let your doctor know right away.

If you have hypothyroidism and it's deemed permanent, you will be medicating with synthetic T4 forever.

How Will Your Treatment Work?

The goal of the synthetic T4 treatment is to get your TSH levels to somewhere in the middle of the normal range and then to keep it there. You'll most likely begin with a low dose (unless your levels were deficient to start with). You'll have your TSH checked via more blood tests about six to eight weeks after starting treatment to look at how your body reacts.

If it's deemed necessary, your doctor will make adjustments to the dose. Keep repeating this process until your TSH is in the normal range. It should be noted that a good doctor will be careful not to give you too high of dosage because excessive doses can place strain on your heart and also increase your risk for osteoporosis.

Excessive amounts of the hormone can also cause a wide range of side effects, like insomnia, shakiness, increased appetite, and heart palpitations.

If you already have any type of coronary artery disease or very bad hypothyroidism, your doctor may begin treatment with a much smaller amount of synthetic T4 and then increase the dosage. This gives all parts of your body time to catch up and adjust to the changes.

Once it seems that you have established the correct dosage, your TSH and T4 levels will be monitored a lot: most likely every six months to a year.

Get ready for a lot of blood tests.

When starting treatment, it may take many weeks before you begin to notice any changes or feel relief.

Most people must stay on this medication forever, but that dosage will change from time to time. If your blood levels ever indicate that the synthetic T4 isn't working as well as it once did or should, your doctor will need to make the dosage adjustments.

Natural Remedies

In some cases, natural remedies are preferred and may actually fit into your lifestyle better.

Let's take a look at some natural things to try.

Selenium

Selenium is said to be an element that actually plays a role in your thyroid hormone metabolism. Some forms of hypothyroidism actually reduce selenium amounts in your body. Some foods that contain selenium are turkey, Brazil nuts, grass-fed beef, and tuna. It has been found that in some cases, supplementing with selenium is effective in helping to balance your T4 levels.

Going Sugar-free

Uh-oh! Nobody wants to hear that they have to break up with sugar. It is said that sugar and processed foods cause inflation in the body. The problem with this is that inflammation actually slows down your body's conversion of T4 into T3, another thyroid hormone.

This makes everything worse.

Also, looking at it from another angle, sugar gives you a short-term energy boost, and getting rid of it may help you balance your depleted energy levels.

Going sugar-free can make your skin appear better and can reduce stress.

Vitamin B

Hypothyroidism can deplete your body's natural vitamin B-12 levels.

A vitamin B-12 supplement may undo some of this damage and replace what has been lost. It can also assist with feeling tired and exhaustion that you experience as a result of hypothyroidism. Hypothyroidism is also known to affect your vitamin B-1 levels. Certain foods such as asparagus, tuna, cheese, peas and beans, sesame seeds, milk, and eggs contain B vitamins.

Probiotics

There's a link between hypothyroidism and small intestine complications. It was discovered that low thyroid levels can bring on gastrointestinal symptoms like diarrhea.

Probiotic supplements contain levels of live beneficial bacteria that are good for your intestines and stomach. You can get probiotics in a pill form or through some food and drink sources such as kombucha, certain cheeses, and yogurt.

Iodine Supplements

Iodine is found in seafood and is an essential nutrient to build the thyroid hormone. Up to a third of the population is deficient in iodine.

Gluten-free diet

Going gluten-free may be a significant pain in the butt, but it was found that many individuals with hypothyroidism also have celiac disease, a digestive disorder.

When gluten is consumed, it triggers an immune response in your small intestines. It has been found that those with hypothyroidism sometimes find some symptom relief after ridding of wheat and other gluten-containing foods from their daily diet.

Keep in mind that going gluten-free is costly. Some prepackaged gluten-free foods are not very health-conscious, as they have high-fat contents to replace the wheat that must be left out.

Herbs

It's believed that herbs are a fantastic approach to aid and strengthen your body's systems.

As with any type of natural or holistic approach, you are recommended and advised to work with your doctor to diagnose your condition and oversee ALL treatment. This includes using herbs. Sometimes, herbs can impact your real success with certain medications, so be sure to do your research and ask your care provider.

Herbs can be taken as dried extracts in the form of powders, capsules, or teas.

They also come in the form of tinctures (alcohol extracts), or glycerites (glycerin extracts). It should be noted that you should not try tinctures if you have any current or past alcoholism issues. Some herbs to try are coleus for low thyroid function, guggul, to support a slow thyroid and bladderwrack, which is also known to support a sluggish thyroid. It should be noted that bladderwrack contains iodine.

Pigs

Doctors will recommend only synthetic thyroxine. But natural extracts containing pig thyroid hormones are out there. They have products that contain both thyroxine and triiodothyronine.

L-tyrosine

To function, your thyroid gland mixes tyrosine and iodine to produce thyroid hormone. L-tyrosine can assist with a tyrosine deficiency.

If you take prescribed thyroid hormone medicine, you should only ingest L-tyrosine under your doctor's supervision.

Please note that you should not take L-tyrosine if you struggle with high blood pressure or show any signs or symptoms of mania.

Medication Tips

Your medication is usually absorbed best on an empty stomach. Be sure that you do not take antacids or any iron supplemental when you are taking medicine because they can interfere with or block the absorption of the synthetic thyroid hormone. Although some factors, such as being pregnant or on other types of medications may affect your need for and dosage of synthetic T4, if you are healthy and taking care of yourself, your dosage should not ever change.

Levothyroxine does not have any side effects when taken, and it is cost-effective. If, for any reason, you do change medication brands, be sure to inform your doctor so he or she can be sure your dosage is the same.

Speaking of brands, **stick with the same one.**

You don't want to confuse your body by overdosing or under-dosing and mixing in different inactive ingredients.

Be sure to not skip any doses or stop taking medicine because you start to feel better. If you do, your symptoms will come back. Again, this is a medicine that usually needs to be taken for the rest of your life.

Please be aware that particular medications, vitamins, and supplements and even some foods may affect your body's ability to absorb the levothyroxine. A high-fiber diet may impact this, or even soy products may affect your body's absorption. Some iron supplements, antacids, and calcium supplements also may affect your medication absorption.

Homeopathy

Homeopathy can be used as a type of therapy to support your hypothyroid condition.

Homeopathic medications for hypothyroidism include Calc-phos., Calc-c., sodium, Thyroidinum, Lapis-alb, Calc-iod., Spong., and Lycopus.

These medicines perform their work on your body where the immunity occurs and works to repair the function that is not operating. These medications are known to help to ease or control the effects of the symptoms of hypothyroidism, and they do not have any side effects. It's said that these homeopathic treatments offer a permanent, but a gradual cure to hypothyroidism.

It should be identified that these homeopathic medications for hypothyroidism are tailored to each person as we are all different and need different things. Thus, a very detailed medical history is necessary before starting any form of homeopathic treatment. A customized homeopathic plan can be put into place to be overseen by your primary care physician.

Exercise and Hypothyroidism

Exercise is essential for those who suffer from hypothyroidism. But, with symptoms that make you sleepy and feel achy, the desire to work out may not be there. Yet, being active will make you feel much better and could make all the difference.

> *"If your condition is well controlled, you should be able to do the same physical activity as someone without a thyroid disorder,"* Stated John C. Morris, MD, professor of medicine and endocrinology at the Mayo Clinic College of Medicine.

So if you're new to exercising or having symptoms that impact your energy and physical well-being, low-impact aerobic exercises will keep the pressure on your joints and muscles low. Coming up, we will further dive depper into exercising with hypothyroidism.

When to See an Endocrinologist

Endocrinology is a medical specialty that involves much more advanced training in your body's endocrine system. The endocrine system includes many of your body's glands and organs that secrete different hormones such as the thyroid, testes, pancreas, and adrenal glands.

Tamara Wexler, MD, Ph.D., an endocrinologist from NYU Langone Health in New York City, suggests anyone diagnosed with hypothyroidism to make an appointment to see an endocrine specialist at least one time when you are first diagnosed with the condition.

This appointment with the endocrinologist will help you to review your current thyroid condition.

Your specialist can help you go over your test results and your individualized treatment plan while answering any questions or tending to any concerns you may have.

"After one or two visits, you may not need to keep seeing him or her," Wexler states.

From here, your primary doctor can generally take over and continue treatment.

There may be other times when it's better to make an appointment to see an endocrinologist.

Specific individuals may have a tough time finding the right type of drugs that best perform for them.

An endocrinologist may be able to better assist you in determining which kind of medication will provide optimal results for you.

If you notice a thyroid lump or nodule, make an appointment with your endocrinologist as soon as possible. Your specialist should examine the bulge. It should be noted that usually, most lumps and bumps on the thyroid are benign, meaning non-cancerous.

Yet, sometimes, they can be indicative of a much larger problem. According to the Cleveland Clinic, about five percent of all thyroid nodules are cancerous.

If you have developed a goiter, which is when a part or all your thyroid gland becomes enlarged, you definitely need to see an endocrinologist. They will assist you in determining the cause and a treatment plan that works best for you.

If you're told that a pituitary gland disorder may be the actual cause of your hypothyroidism, this too requires a trip to the endocrinologist.

Your pituitary gland, along with your hypothalamus, is located at the bottom or base of your brain. The liver oversees and regulates your body's production of thyroid hormone. The pituitary gland is the cause of hypothyroidism. But, in some individuals, the pituitary gland can fail to or slow down the release of the thyrotropin-releasing hormone, also known as TRH.

In turn, this stimulates your thyroid to produce thyroid hormone. Due to how complicated this disorder is, seeking the help of an endocrinologist is in your best interest to receive the best care.

If you're already pregnant or planning to try to become pregnant, seek out advice from your endocrinologist. They can give you sound advice in regard to how pregnancy will affect your thyroid condition. Pregnancy will, no doubt, alter your hormone levels a great deal. Thus, during this time, your thyroid levels are monitored by an endocrinologist.

Sometimes, for some women, they will need anywhere from 25 to 50 percent more thyroid hormone while pregnant, due to the baby taking it from the mother.

https://www.webmd.com/women/guide/low-thyroid-treatment#1

https://www.medicalnewstoday.com/articles/1637 29#symptoms

https://www.healthline.com/health/hypothyroidis m/five-natural-remedies-for-hypothyroidism#gluten-free-diet

https://www.webmd.com/women/features/exercis es-underactive-thyroid#1

https://www.everydayhealth.com/hs/healthy-living-with-hypothyroidism/see-an-endocrinologist/

http://pennstatehershey.adam.com/content.aspx?p roductid=107&pid=33&gid=000093

https://www.wellinghomeopathy.com/treatment-hypothyroid/#Homeopathic_treatment_forHypoth yroid

CHAPTER 4

LIVING WITH HYPOTHYROIDISM

Hypothyroidism will have some type of impact on your social and emotional life. Having a healthy support system is one of the many ways to assist with this. Staying active is very important for both your physical and mental health.

Being aware of your mental health state, and having healthy habits with a lifestyle that best serves you is paramount.

Emotional

Keeping up with and managing having hypothyroidism can elicit a wide range of emotions. You may have almost felt bipolar at times as you can feel sadness, anger, and frustration all at once or one after the other.

Missing out on sleep, having a sedentary lifestyle, and not getting the proper nutrients in your diet can make these emotions and feelings worse. You need to keep up with yourself and tune in to these feelings and find their source.

Sorting through these emotions can prove to be complicated. Sometimes therapy can help because it's said that depression and anxiety can go hand in hand with hypothyroidism.

Therapy and medication can help you to cope with mental health complications.

Thyroid and Stress

Many studies show that stress may actually trigger or make hypothyroidism even worse. Human and animal studies have shown that stress can affect your immune system via your endocrine and nervous systems. These alterations can contribute to thyroid deficiency.

When your body is under stress, you resort to a "fight or flight" mode and course of action. Your body does this to remove any attention from healing and digestion and to pump adrenaline to prepare yourself to survive the threat it perceives.

This stress contributes to the inadequate production of thyroid hormones.

Ways to Relieve Stress

There are many ways and beneficial practices that you can take on to reduce stress.

Meditation can assist with improving your focus, boosting hormones, and relieving anxiety.

Yoga can help to calm the body, mind, and nervous system.

Healthy sleeping habits, like getting at least eight hours of sleep each night, can make a huge difference.

Praying and getting involved in spiritual practices can reduce stress levels.

Get a massage.

Focusing on yourself in the form of journaling and staying mindful of your thoughts and feelings.

And as we've already discussed, go exercise.

Physical

Taking care of yourself is also a big part of handling hypothyroidism. Unexplained weight gain is a very unwelcome symptom of the condition but the good news is losing weight is in your control.

We're already aware that weight gain and the difficulty of losing weight is there.

Exercise Principals

Getting yourself moving and your heart rate up, for at least thirty minutes five times a week, is a significant component of your health, especially with hypothyroidism.

Daily movement and exercise can help:

- Speed up your metabolism
- Reduce fatigue and muscle pain
- Curb your appetite
- Increase your serotonin levels,
- Bring down unhealthy blood glucose levels
- Lower your cortisol (stress) levels.

Regular workouts actually can help to combat how tired and lethargic you are from hypothyroidism.

Exercise also makes for much better sleep, which may be fragmented as a result of the condition.

Your mood will be elevated from getting enough exercise, and your endorphins, also known as "feel-good hormones," will get flowing. One exciting thing that exercise can do is increase your bone density, which is usually affected by hypothyroidism.

Working out speeds up your metabolism.

This is important to keep note because when dealing with hypothyroidism, your metabolism slows down, causing weight gain. Exercising can be used to help catalyze metabolism and start your weight loss journey..

Fitness trackers are an excellent suggestion to motivate you and to encourage you to get moving.

You can also look into a fitness program accessible on a cell phone app or video for some workout ideas and plans.

What Type of Exercise Should You Do?

For those with hypothyroidism, the best type of exercise depends on your health.

Your preferred type of activity is also essential. Usually, if your condition is under control and well-monitored and you are in good health, you can exercise in any way that you see fit.

Low- Impact Exercises

If you're starting out or haven't exercised in a long time, you will want to start nice and slow. If you're not feeling too high either, opting for some low-impact exercises will allow yourself time and opportunity to build up endurance and strength.

Some low-impact options include:

- Walking
- Bike riding
- Indoor cycling
- Strength training with bodyweight
- Stair climbing
- Yoga
- Water aerobics
- Swimming
- Dancing

Mixing these up will keep things fresh and will help to avoid boredom. You can work towards building up the intensity of your workouts as your body gets stronger.

High-Impact Exercises

If you are already in decent shape, you can opt for some high-impact exercises such as:

- Jogging and Running
- Jumping Jacks
- HIIT (High-Intensity Interval Training)
- Jumping Rope
- Weight training

Two yoga poses for hypothyroidism

Two primary poses pulled from healthline.com, that may assist with hypothyroidism are the supported shoulder stand and the plow pose.

Supported Shoulder Stand

The supported shoulder stand pose will put your body upside down, which is called an inversion in the yogi world.

Inversions are said to increase the blood flow to your throat, which can help to stimulate your thyroid gland.

To make a supported shoulder stand, a person should:

- Lie down flat on the back
- Place a folded towel or blanket under the shoulders to support them
- Bring the shoulders to the edge of the sheet while resting the head on the mat
- Place the arms on either side with palms facing down
- Press arms and back into the floor
- Breathe in and lift legs up at a right angle
- Breathe out and lift legs up, pushing up onto the shoulders
- Push hands into the lower back to support the hips
- Keep the stomach pulled in, so the core is strong
- Hold the body and legs in a straight line up from the shoulders
- Keep the chin tucked into the chest
- Breathe deep three times
- Lower the legs back down slow, keeping the core engaged

The Plow Pose

The Plow Pose is also said to stimulate the thyroid.

To do the Plow Pose, a person should begin in the same way as for a shoulder stand.

Rather than holding the legs up in a straight line from the shoulders, they should:

- Bring the legs right over and behind their head
- Rest their toes on the floor behind their head
- Keep their lower back supported with their hands throughout
- Breathe deep three times
- Bring the legs back above the head
- Lower the legs back to the floor, keeping the core engaged

If your hypothyroidism isn't under control or has not been diagnosed yet, be cautious of going extreme when exercising. Undiagnosed hypothyroidism can be challenging on your cardiac health if your thyroid hormones aren't regulated.

Exercise Guidelines

Figuring out the proper amount of exercise for you can prove to be rather tricky.

To see noticeable health benefits for your hypothyroidism, adults should be trying to incorporate five days of training at least an hour.

This can include moderate aerobic exercise, such as playing basketball or tennis, walking at a brisk pace, water aerobics, or bicycling.

Some vigorous aerobic activities, such as swimming laps, jogging, bicycling, and running, are more experienced.

As earlier mentioned, you should also be working on moderate- to high-intensity muscle-strengthening exercises and weightlifting that incorporate all your major muscle groups.

Strength training in hypothyroidism is essential because muscle mass will help to fire up your metabolism that is slowed down as a result of the condition.

Make sure that you have proper nutrition while exercising. If you're trying to go big or go home, bump your moderate aerobic activity to around five hours per week and your vigorous aerobic exercise to about two hours and 30 minutes per week.

It's essential to talk to your doctor if your hypothyroidism symptoms aren't improving as a result of exercising or getting worse.

Once your hypothyroidism symptoms are under control, and hormone levels are regulated, including exercise back into your routine is encouraged.

Staying Motivated

When you have hypothyroidism, it's possible that you can get bored with exercise.

Here are some tips that may help you maintain your motivation while exercising.

Hire A Personal Trainer

A trainer may be able to put together and design an exercise plan that fits your needs and stays sensitive to your hypothyroidism. They can also show you the safest way to perform exercise movements to avoid injury.

Make sure to communicate about your condition so they can cater your training.

Personal Trainers can provide motivation, as many of us work harder when we know that others are observing, especially coaching. Having a personal trainer with you can be a form of encouragement to actually work out. With a personal trainer, you can set fitness goals that go with your road to a healthier functioning thyroid.

Staying accountable to a personal trainer can help you stay on track when you struggle to stick with a routine or program.You won't be able to use excuses to get out of a workout. It's a lot more challenging to skip the gym when you know that your trainer is sitting there waiting.

Another benefit to hiring a personal trainer could be that the gym is too intimidating. Learning how to use the machines, barbells, and free weights can be confusing at first.

Even bodyweight exercises can prove to be challenging to figure out if you don't know what you're doing. Having a personal trainer there with you brings on confidence that you are performing the tasks and navigating the gym as you should. Even if you only use a trainer in the beginning, after a couple sessions, you will feel much more confident in the gym. It's said that having confidence while working out can bring on a stronger sense of self-confidence and self-efficacy. This can assist in sticking with your exercise program in the long run.

Working out should be fun. With a personal trainer, they can help you to tap into that fun aspect. Sometimes, they can incorporate group or buddy workouts with others. By making exercise more social, you have a way to take your mind off of what you are actually doing.

Work Out with Friends

Getting moving with your friends will help you to stay committed and show up!

It's almost like you are tricking yourself into working out for another person. It's also an excellent way to keep distracted from the actual act of working out, as you can talk to each other while being motivated. It's a win-win! You may even make some new friends along the way.

Listen to Music While Working Out

Music takes your mind off of the actual act of working out. There are many playlists and mixes out there, so you can find something to your liking. The tunes will lift your spirits and keep you bumping and pressing onward through your workout.

Remember, exercise is so very critical to your health with hypothyroidism. We spent a lot of time discussing it to ensure that you incorporate it into your lifestyle.

Recommended Hypothyroidism Work Out

Igor Klibanov, a well-known personal trainer in Canada and founder of "Fitness Solutions Plus" recommends a workout plan that consists of both cardio and strength training with 6 simple exercises:

One-legged Deadlift:

Stand on one leg while holding onto something for balance (not for support). Keep one hand relaxed in front of your thigh. Push your hips as far back as you can, until your hand touches the ground. Come back up. You should feel this in the glutes (the butt muscles). The back should not curve; it should stay straight but does not have to be upright.

Squats

Stand up straight and then bend at your hips and knees till you're in a sitting position. Go down all the way. (Klibanov says it's a myth that this will damage your knees if you have healthy knees, begin with.).

Overhead Press

Raise a pair of dumbbells to shoulder height. Turn your arms, so they're facing forward. Lift the dumbbells up until your elbows are straight. Then lower them back down to your shoulders.

Lat pull-down or similar vertical pull move

Grab a pull-down bar with an overhand grip (palms facing away) and pull it down to your collarbone. Keep your back straight, and make sure the bar travels as close to your face as possible.

Push-ups or similar push movements.

Put both hands on the floor, shoulder-width apart. Feet should be pushed out and together. Bend your elbows and shoulders until you're close to the ground. If push-ups are hard, do the same thing either with your hands on a table (while feet stay on the ground) or a wall.

Rowing or similar horizontal pull move.

Sit on a rowing machine with your hands holding the handle that's attached to the cable. Keep your back straight and lean back about 10 to15 degrees. Pull the cord back until it touches your mid-stomach. Then release under control.

Start with 15 reps of each exercise and work up to 20. "Most people with joint problems find these to be easy on the joints," Klibanov says. When you're starting out, it may take you 15 to 20 minutes to complete your routine. A good, eventual goal: Work up to three sets of 15 to 20 reps, which should take about 40 to 45 minutes.

"Schedule aerobic exercise three to four times a week and strength training with these moves two to three days a week" Klibanov recommends.

Doing so can get you on the right track to losing weight and feeling better."

Eating Right

Nourishing yourself while dealing with hypothyroidism can be challenging. You can consider a nutritionist to help you maintain a healthy weight and eat in such a way that supports your thyroid condition.

We will later discuss more what to and not to consume.

Social

It's much more manageable and straightforward to stay on track with your hypothyroidism if you have the support and encouragement of loved ones and friends.

While you're struggling with the many stressors and symptoms of hypothyroidism, support from friends, your doctor, family, and others can help with stress, anxiety, and the emotional ups and downs that come with the condition.

"Having an under-active thyroid shouldn't keep you from any activities of daily living," stated Tamara Wexler, MD Ph.D.

When you are diagnosed with the condition, your blood tests and dosage adjustments are made at about six-week intervals, and while the doctor is trying to find the proper dosage, it may take three or more months to begin to see improvements.

This means that you may have a few grouchy and difficult months where you may need some support. Leaning on others will prove to be very beneficial.

Getting out and interacting with others can be a very healthy distraction from your hypothyroidism. Do not miss out on others because of your condition!

Your Family

It should be mentioned that if you're diagnosed with hypothyroidism, you need to tell those that you're related to the diagnosis because hypothyroidism does not run in the family.

Your family members will most likely want to get a blood test as well. Your family needs to know and understand that you're going through some pretty tough hormonal changes that can affect the way you feel.

Offline and Online Support Groups

Besides reaching out to your loved ones and getting them involved, you may want to join a thyroid support group. There are even online groups if that better serves your comfortability or availability.

You must go into it with an open mind and with patience as it may take a few tries until you find a group that meets your needs.

If you're a mother with hypothyroidism, you may be interested in finding other moms with the same condition. That way, they may be able to relate better and offer tips and solutions to issues that they have encountered in their daily lives.

The bottom line here is that connecting with other individuals who empathize and sympathize while understanding your changes and symptoms show that you are not alone.

You may also find tips and some new information on your condition.

Stay Involved

You must stay involved in your entire course of treatment. It's important to always get a copy of your thyroid blood results.

With this documentation, you'll be able to follow along and work alongside your doctor to figure out where your thyroid levels are when you are feeling the best. For some, they think best at the lower end of the normal TSH range, which puts them right at around 1.0.

Some other people may feel the best in the middle of the field, and some like to be towards the higher end. Where you think the best is different from others and finding that level is a critical part of taking control of your hypothyroidism.

It should be mentioned that if you feel like your regular doctor is not able to find that level where you feel your best, seeing an endocrinologist is always an option, even for a second opinion.

Your doctor is your partner in your journey with hypothyroidism.

https://www.healthline.com/health/yoga-for-thyroid#yoga-poses

https://www.everydayhealth.com/hs/healthy-living-with-hypothyroidism/get-support/

https://www.medicalnewstoday.com/articles/320744#beneficial-yoga-poses

CHAPTER 5

EATING WELL: MEAL PLANS ANDNUTRITION TIPS

You were diagnosed with hypothyroidism, and now you find out that you need to change some things about the way you eat. These types of changes are never dull.

Those individuals diagnosed with hypothyroidism need to be prepared to find and learn about foods that they should eat more of as well as foods that they should avoid.

It should be noted that there is no specific diet or way of eating for those who struggle with hypothyroidism. Consuming a low-fat diet with a right and steady balance of fruits, vegetables, dairy, lean protein, poultry, fish and lean meats, and whole grains is a great strategy and the general way to go when combating this condition.

You can't go wrong with eating clean and healthy!

Calories

You want to be sure that you are portioning out and balancing your calorie intake throughout your day. Speaking of calories, watching what you eat will aid in preventing weight gain.

Because hypothyroidism slows down your metabolism, making it sluggish, it is quite easy for you to gain weight. Managing that calorie intake plays an important role.

Your basal metabolic rate (BMR) involves calculating the calories that your body burns to keep you functioning and alive.

BMR actually is engaged in anywhere between fifty to eighty percent of all the calories that you consume. The rest is accounted for by exercise, digestion, and healthy body functions.

When taking hypothyroidism into account, it varies on how much your thyroid problem slows down your own personal BMR. If someone does not have any thyroid due to surgical removal, they are looking at a 40% percent drop in BMR.

On the flip side, if someone's thyroid is functioning, they are around 6%.

That's a vast and significant difference.

For a few individuals, this drop doesn't make a big difference, especially if they take their thyroid medication daily. That person does not struggle with bodyweight problems any more than someone living without any thyroid problems.

But for those who let their hypothyroidism go untreated, this can cut down the number of calories that their own bodies burn in a typical day by more than three hundred calories.

This hinders weight loss.

Someone who doesn't have any thyroid problems can drop much more weight than those who have hypothyroidism, especially when it is not treated.

Having mentioned this, there are three particular diets that you may want to look into.

The Autoimmune Diet

This autoimmune diet (AIP) is considered to be a modified paleo diet. It focuses on eliminating some inflammatory foods and potential allergens such as grains, dairy, legumes, nuts, eggs, seeds, nightshades, sugar and sweeteners, alcohol, and several food additives.

It's said that autoimmune diets may quiet down the symptoms in those people with Hashimoto's thyroiditis, an autoimmune disease that attacks the thyroid.

We discussed what the no's are for AIP, but let's take a look at what you can have.

While on an autoimmune diet, you can indulge in many types of meat and veggies. Coconut products, such as coconut oil, are great, along with olive oil and non-dairy fermented foods.

These include:

- Kombucha
- Non-dairy kefir
- Fermented veggies
- Red wine vinegar
- Apple Cider Vinegar

- Balsamic Vinegar

In addition, herbs, honey, maple syrup, gelatin from grass-fed beef, and arrowroot starch are all acceptable on an AIP diet.

While fruits are usually controversial on AIP's, they can be consumed.

The Anti-Inflammatory Diet

Inflammation can impact the autoimmune response in those with Hashimoto's thyroiditis and make it worse.

So, an eating plan that works off of anti-inflammatory foods can benefit these people.

Berries are a great anti-inflammatory food. Although they are small fruits, they are chock full of vitamins, minerals, and fiber. Blueberries, strawberries, raspberries, and blackberries all contain antioxidants known as anthocyanins, which may aid in reducing inflammation, can boost your immune system and reduce your risk of contracting cardiovascular disease.

Make sure to get your greens as well. Broccoli, kale, Brussels sprouts, and cauliflower all are known as cruciferous veggies, meaning that they have a lot of anti-inflammatory effects.

Avocados, while packed with fiber, magnesium, and potassium, also offer anti-inflammatory compounds and can also reduce your risk of cancer.

Green tea is very high in anti-inflammatory properties that are also known to boost your immune system.

Consuming types of fatty fish are also known to be great. They are a fabulous protein source and have lots of healthy fats and omegas. Some of the best types of fish are salmon, herring, anchovies, sardines, and mackerel.

Both bell peppers and chili peppers contain antioxidants and vitamin C, and these have amazing anti-inflammatory effects. Bell peppers are known to provide the antioxidant, quercetin, which fights against any inflammation.

Chili peppers have sinapic acid and ferulic acid in them, and these acids are said to slow down the effects of aging and reduce inflammation.

Grapes are packed with anthocyanins, which reduce inflammation and are great to snack on.

Mushrooms, yes, mushrooms, are also helpful in this regard. With so many different types around, mushrooms only have a few that can be eaten. They contain selenium, copper, and even the B vitamins that will assist with being sleepy. Mushrooms are rich in phenols and some other types of antioxidants, which reduce any inflammation.

Turmeric is a spice for cooking (found in Indian cuisines and dishes) and contains curcumin, a proven anti-inflammatory.

Extra virgin olive oil (EVOO) has been linked to the ability to reduce the risk of a heart attack, heart disease, and even brain cancer. It also goes down in the books as a very effective inflammation reducer.

Cherries also contain some anthocyanin and catechins, which fight against any inflammation in your body and help to boost your immune system while fighting off any sickness.

Tomatoes can decrease inflammation. They contain lycopene, an antioxidant that is known for its anti-inflammatory properties. They also contain a large amount of vitamin C and potassium, providing your immune system with a nice boost.

Dark chocolate, and cocoa contain tons of

antioxidants that reduce any inflammation in your body. Flavanol is present in dark chocolate and handles this sweet little perk. You should be sure to choose dark chocolate comprising at least 70% cocoa for optimal benefits.

The Elimination Diet

If you remove certain foods and then reintroduce them, you can figure out rather which foods elicit reactions and problems for you.

Elimination diets only go on for five or six weeks and can be used to figure out what foods may cause nasty symptoms. You may even get rid of some bloating, gas, constipation, diarrhea, and nausea.

Once you do figure out which type of food your body may not tolerate well, you can remove it from your diet and stop consuming it to fix any problems or issues that it may have caused.

There are tons of different forms of elimination diets, but they all incorporate you removing specific types of foods that you once ate and then re-introducing them.

With elimination diets, it should be noted that if you are aware or even suspect that you have a food allergy, do not try an elimination diet unless you are under doctor supervision.

Reintroducing a food allergen into your diet can have some terrible reactions such as hives, rashes, swelling, and even difficulty breathing.

Deficiencies

Several deficiencies can contribute to your hypothyroidism.

Iodine

Iodine is necessary for thyroid hormone production. Your thyroid gland won't be able to produce ample thyroid hormone if it doesn't get enough iodine. Iodized salt is one way to ensure avoidance of iodine deficiency. Those people who eat very clean may actually lack iodized salt in their diet and may need to be cognizant of this.

Healthy individuals will choose sea salt, which contains very little iodine, and consume very little if any, processed food rich in iodized salt.

Iron

Iron helps your body make red blood cells and is also a massive player in TSH production. Somewhere around 43 percent of those with hypothyroidism also suffer from iron-deficiency anemia. Iron is involved in the proper production of your thyroid hormones. When you're deficient in iron, this affects the proper function of your thyroid.

Without iron, anyone struggling with hypothyroidism can be hindered when it comes to healing the thyroid. The main reason is that iron plays a significant role in regulating your immune system.

Selenium

Selenium is a mineral that assists your thyroid in creating thyroid hormone. Selenium deficiency is rare, but those individuals who have had gastric bypass surgery or who struggle with Crohn's disease or kidney problems may be deficient in selenium.

Zinc

Zinc is a massive component in seafood, such as oysters and shellfish. Zinc is also present in beef and other red meats. Non-meat forms of zinc like grains, nuts, and legumes, are not available for absorption by your body because they are bound with phytic acid, which prevents this absorption.

So, those who are vegan, vegetarian, or don't eat fish may struggle with a zinc deficiency altogether.

This is problematic because zinc works with vitamins A and E to make the thyroid hormone and to convert T4 to T3.

Zinc is also known to assist in other hormone activities, such as growth hormones, insulin, and function of your immune system.

Copper

It has been proven that your body's T3 and T4 levels of your thyroid hormones go hand in hand with your body's blood copper levels. When you experience low blood copper levels, your thyroid hormone levels go down as well.

This can impact your thyroid function. Copper is present in your drinking water, but you can wind up being deficient if you supplement it with zinc at the same time. This is because zinc actually binds to the same cell receptor sites, and the zinc can overpower the copper.

Tyrosine

Tyrosine is an amino acid located in meats, fish, dairy products, nuts, eggs, oats, wheat, and beans. Tyrosine is involved in the making of your thyroid hormones.

Magnesium

Magnesium is essential to your whole body as it is involved in about three hundred enzymatic reactions. In cases of bad hypothyroidism, your blood pressure gets higher as a direct result of the loss of plasticity of your body's blood vessels. Magnesium regulates your blood pressure by preventing excessive constrictions of the blood vessels.

Magnesium is located in chlorophyll and is found in large amounts in green vegetables, grains, and nuts.

A Quick Glance at Goitrogens

Some types of foods that you eat contain substances called goitrogens. Goitrogens stop your thyroid gland from absorbing iodine, which your thyroid relies on to function.

Some foods that contain goitrogens are cruciferous vegetables such as bok choy, kale, broccoli, cauliflower.

Some other foods that contain them are peanuts, soy, turnips, grapeseed, and cassava. It's essential to note that those with hypothyroidism don't need to cut out or avoid goitrogenic foods as they are not a massive issue for everyone, and if they are a problem for you, there is an easy fix. If you cook these foods, the healing process and the cooking actually deactivates most of the goitrogens.

Radiation and Toxins

Some foods and products have been proven to affect your thyroid functioning, and you should stay away from them, as they can be viewed as toxins to you. These include unfiltered tap water (even for bathing also) as they may contain heavy metals and pesticides.

Also, on the list are inorganic meats and fairy because they may have hormone and antibiotic residues. Some fish may have mercury, and because most cleaning products are harsh, it is a good idea to keep your distance. Dental X-rays are done via radiation, and cigarettes and fire retardants may contain harmful chemicals. Fluoride should also be avoided.

Hypothyroid Meal Plan

Now that you have an idea of which foods to go for and which to avoid, it is time to put it together and start determining what to eat throughout the day so you can build that grocery list.

Going with a whole food diet with appropriate amounts of fats and protein, coupled with plenty of nutritious vegetables, will work wonders for your body.

Here is an example of what a few days of eating should look like:

Example #1

Breakfast (Remember to wait at least 1-2 hours after taking your medication to eat)

3 egg omelets with spinach, mushrooms, tomato, and avocado on the side.
Served with green tea or kombucha

Lunch

Grilled chicken diced over a baby green mixed salad with onions, sliced red bell pepper, chopped apple, and brazil nut parmesan balsamic vinaigrette dressing.

Dinner

Baked salmon, corn on the cob, and asparagus with a spinach cranberry salad with bacon

Snacks:

Celery sticks with almond butter, apple slices, and peanut butter, or thin slices of deli meat and crackers.

Example #2

Breakfast

Oatmeal with apples and cinnamon

Lunch

Quinoa Salad with tomatoes, cucumbers, and feta cheese

Dinner

Chicken and Broccoli Stir fry, cottage cheese

Snacks

Celery and carrots with hummus

Example #3

Breakfast
Plain Greek yogurt with granola and berries

Lunch
Grilled chicken salad topped with walnuts and pumpkin seeds with an extra virgin olive oil and vinegar dressing.

Dinner
Beef fajitas with peppers and onions served with green tea.

Snacks
Protein bars and apple

Example #4

Breakfast
Quinoa and blueberry bake

Lunch
Turkey and cheese sandwich on gluten-free bread

Dinner
Rotisserie chicken served with black beans and rice.

Snacks
Banana

Peanut butter and jelly crackers

https://www.precisionnutrition.com/hypothyroidism-diet-plan

https://drbrighten.com/thyroid-foods-and-one-day-thyroid-meal-plan/

CHAPTER 6

LISTEN TO YOUR BODY: COMPLICATIONS OF UNTREATED HYPOTHYROIDISM

Hypothyroidism is not a condition that will go away in a day. Hypothyroidism requires treatment, and then a lot of monitoring to deliver the best results possible. If it's left untreated, some myriad other issues and problems may arise that could impact your health. Catching the condition and its side effects and risk factors early, along with constant intervention, is the key to living a happy and productive life with hypothyroidism.

Birth Defects

Becoming pregnant with an untreated thyroid disorder opens up the door for quite a few possible complications. Having hypothyroidism that is not treated may give your baby a much more significant risk of experiencing birth defects than a baby born with a mother who doesn't have thyroid problems.

Infants born from women with untreated thyroid problems and issues may be susceptible to development issues. They run the risk of mental issues because the baby will not be getting enough thyroid hormones which is important for baby brain development. So it's incredibly important to catch the condition and treat it as quickly as possible to prevent any unwanted issues.

Right after birth, a baby's thyroid levels will typically be checked right away.

Cardiovascular problems

Your thyroid hormone level can impact your cardiovascular health. As a result of letting hypothyroidism go untreated, you may encounter a slow or weakened pulse, or even abnormal heartbeats.

Hypothyroidism can lead to your body retaining

fluid. When this happens, it can lead to hypertension. Hypertension is having high blood pressure, which can result in your heart not pumping enough blood. Worst case scenario, it can lead to a heart attack or congestive heart failure.

Unknown to many, when your body retains this fluid, it's a significant reason and explanation for weight gain. This type of weight gain comes off, looking puffier. Your feet, ankles, and face can seem puffy.

Hypothyroidism also puts your cardiac system at risk by increasing your lipid levels. These are your cholesterol and triglyceride levels. Your lipids, in excess, can cause a fatty lining on your artery walls. This condition is referred to as atherosclerosis.

It was also found that being deficient in the thyroid hormones can decrease the volume of blood that's forced out of your heart by your heart pumping by anywhere from 30 to 50 percent. When you experience low T3 levels, this can send you into heart failure. It's a relief to know that most cardiac problems that result from hypothyroidism can be medicated and treated with the proper medication.

Nervous system complications

Hypothyroidism can impact your nervous system by bringing weakness to your muscles or damage to your nerves. These problems can illicit difficulty breathing, trouble speaking, problems walking, hoarseness in your voice, or pain in your feet or hands. You may even encounter carpal tunnel syndrome.

Fertility Issues

Hypothyroidism reduces fertility in both men and women. Your thyroid hormones, produced by your thyroid gland, are known to regulate your sex hormones metabolism. These sex hormones are what control and oversee the creation of sperm in males and eggs in females.

Women

It's been proven that it's three times as likely for women with hypothyroidism to experience menstrual issues. Having a heavy flow one cycle and then very light flow the next is indicative of this.

Also, having irregular cycles is the most common symptom. This means that there is no clear pattern of when you will get your next period. You may even be going months without a period. It should be noted that women with autoimmune thyroid disorder are much more likely to encounter infertility.

Through many studies, it's been determined that your thyroid hormone is a critical player in the correct development and implantation of your eggs. Studies have shown that infertility impacts almost half of the women who struggle with Hashimoto's thyroiditis based on their low thyroid function and autoimmune disease.

Men

A healthy and functioning thyroid gland is essential for male reproductive health. The proper amount of men's thyroid hormones will determine the fate of their fertility. T3 and T4 are both known to be essential to the proper development and function of your testes.

In men, hypothyroidism goes along with erectile dysfunction, decreased libido, and abnormal sperm shape. Men with hypothyroidism often also have low levels of testosterone.

Men's testosterone levels are destined to be much

lower if their thyroid is not producing enough thyroid hormone. This, in turn, means that their sperm count will also be much lower. On the opposite side, their testicles may even be more significant.

The T3 hormone is essential for testicles to mature and for testosterone to be produced. If your T3 levels are way too low, you will not be producing enough testosterone to be a fertile man.

Why Does Your Thyroid Gland Affect Sperm Morphology?

Sperm morphology is the shape and size of your sperm. To be short and to the point, you need the thyroid hormone for your sperm to have a functioning cytoskeleton. The sperm cytoskeleton is a structure that yields mechanical support to your sperm. This allows the sperm to be able to move onward while keeping its shape.

When you treat your condition with the synthetic T4, also known as levothyroxine, this will balance out your male testosterone levels and improve your sperm morphology and motility.

If you struggle with hypothyroidism as a man, you

may have problems with your semen's density and volume.

Men can reverse any fertility issues brought on by thyroid problems once they get the thyroid gland back to function via treatment and medication.

Pregnancy complications

It's well known that hypothyroidism can cause many pregnancy issues. It can increase your risk of having a miscarriage. It can also bring on many other complications, such as preeclampsia or even preterm birth.

This is one of the reasons why it's so essential for you to keep your doctor informed every step of the way from when you are planning to begin trying to become pregnant all the way through the delivery of that baby. This will ensure that proper treatment is provided every step of the way since medication will need to be adjusted throughout the pregnancy.

If you don't tend to your thyroid issues before becoming pregnant, you're opening the doors to many complications.

Keep in mind that a developing baby will demand a

lot from your body, which can lead to a new onset of the thyroid condition or make your current hypothyroidism case worse.

It has been found that your risk of having a miscarriage may doubled if you are hypothyroid compared to a female who doesn't suffer from a thyroid issue.

Renal complications

The term renal refers to your kidneys. Severe cases of hypothyroidism can even make a significant impact on your kidney function. Brought on by decreased blood flow to your organs. When this happens, you may not be able to excrete water and fluids or absorb sodium from the foods you eat. As a result, your sodium levels in your blood may be low.

Treating your case of hypothyroidism can reverse these renal complications. Yet, it is important to note that your recovery may take much longer if low thyroid hormone levels stick around for some time.

Mental health issues

As stated, depression can pronounce itself early in cases of hypothyroidism. Depression can become more severe over time. Hypothyroidism can also cause mental functioning to slow down.

There was one study conducted that was published in March of 2015 in the journal Endocrine Research.

In this study, individuals with subclinical hypothyroidism were assessed for depression at random, were assigned to be given a placebo or a thyroid hormone. Twelve weeks later, depression improved very much in the thyroid hormone group. But, in the placebo group, depression didn't change much.

This means that treating hypothyroidism is useful in assisting and managing the depression that can go with it. Even if you have no idea that your case of hypothyroidism is having any effect on your mental or emotional health, you may notice a huge change once you begin treatment. You may start to feel more like yourself, more motivated to make things, happier, freer and less weighed down, or a sense of refreshment.

Goiter

A goiter presents itself when your thyroid gland is stimulated while trying very hard to produce more thyroid hormones. This causes the liver to become more prominent, and thus, a goiter is formed.

Although goiters are not painful or uncomfortable, they can impact your appearance and make it very difficult to swallow or even breathe.

"Your endocrine system works in feedback loops," notes Tracy S. Tylee, MD, an endocrinologist at the University of Washington Medical Center in Seattle.

> *"Your brain tells your thyroid how much thyroid hormone to make, and it monitors your thyroid hormone levels to determine this."*

> *"To stimulate your thyroid, your brain creates a hormone called the thyroid-stimulating hormone (TSH). If your thyroid hormone level is low, your brain will make more TSH in an attempt to make your thyroid work harder."*

A goiter will present itself when *"the brain is hammering the thyroid, trying to get more thyroid hormone out of it,"* says Dr. Tylee. *"When that happens, the thyroid gets bigger and bigger as it's trying to make more thyroid hormone."*

> *"A goiter isn't usually dangerous or uncomfortable,"* says Tylee,

"but it's often an early warning sign of thyroid dysfunction — even before your thyroid hormone levels fall below normal — and it's a sign that you should get your TSH level checked."

Sometimes, a goiter can even lead to thyroid surgery.

Types of thyroid surgery

There are many different types of thyroid surgery. The most common types are a lobectomy, total thyroidectomy, and subtotal thyroidectomy.

Lobectomy

A lobectomy happens when your doctor decides to only take one of the two lobes of your thyroid gland. On occasion, a nodule, swelling, or inflammation will impact only half of your thyroid gland.

In this case, a lobectomy is opted for, and your doctor will remove only one of the two lobes. Usually, if the procedure is a success, the part of your thyroid gland that winds up being left behind should function. Many follow-ups will be done to check up on and ensure this.

Subtotal Thyroidectomy

A subtotal thyroidectomy happens when your doctor removes your whole thyroid gland but actually leaves behind a minimal amount of your thyroid tissue.

This actually will save some of your thyroid function.

When you undergo this type of surgical procedure, you're at risk of developing hypothyroidism, if you don't already have it.

Total thyroidectomy

When you undergo total thyroidectomy, your doctor will remove your entire thyroid, as well as your thyroid tissue. This surgery is the only option that you may have if you have thyroid swelling, thyroid nodules, or thyroid inflammation.

How is Thyroid Surgery Performed?

If you need to have a procedure performed, the thyroid surgery will be done in a hospital setting, as it is a strict procedure. You will most likely be instructed to not eat or drink anything after midnight the night before your thyroid surgery.

Upon arrival at the hospital, you'll be told to check-in. You'll most likely be sent into an area to get prepped for surgery. They will have you remove your clothing and slip into a hospital gown. Hospital gowns are fashionable. A nurse will set you up with an IV into either your wrist or your arm. This IV will provide you with medicine and fluids to keep you safe and comfortable during the whole procedure.

Before your surgery, your surgeon will come to see you, conduct a brief examination, and answer any questions you may have. They can ease any concerns as well. You'll also be introduced to your anesthesiologist.

An anesthesiologist administers the medication while you are under during the whole procedure.

When the time comes for your surgery, medical staff will transport you into the operating room on a gurney. Your anesthesiologist will administer medicine into your IV to put you under. You may feel cold or a sting as the medication is delivered into your body.

Your surgeon will most likely make an incision in your skin over the area your thyroid gland is on your neck. From here, they will remove all parts of the organ that's necessary. It's an intricate procedure due to the size and the many nerves surrounding it.

Upon waking up, you will find yourself in the recovery room. The hospital staff will be ensuring that you are comfortable and will be checking your vitals and giving you medication. From here, you will most likely be kept for a few days to be monitored.

Robotic Thyroidectomy

Another type of thyroid surgery is known as a robotic thyroidectomy. It's a procedure in which your surgeon can remove specific parts of your thyroid through an axillary incision. This means that he or she will go through the armpit. Your doctor can also do this, or through your mouth.

Because this is invasive, you can most likely get back to your typical daily activities the day after your surgery. But it's recommended that you wait for up to ten days, or until your doctor gives you the go-ahead, to partake in any form of strenuous activity. This means no high-impact exercise for this period.

Your throat will likely feel sore for many days following the procedure. You may be able to give yourself an over-the-counter pain medication to help.

Ibuprofen or acetaminophen will work fine in this case.

If your pain is not relieved with these mediations, your doctor may be able to prescribe you some narcotic pain medication.

After you undergo this type of surgery, you can develop hypothyroidism if you do not already suffer from it. If this does happen, your doctor will prescribe you some kind of levothyroxine to balance your thyroid hormone levels. This will make many adjustments to get the dosage right for you.

Peripheral Neuropathy

Peripheral neuropathy occurs in your body when you leave hypothyroidism left unattended for an extended period. This can damage your peripheral nerves. Peripheral nerves are the nerves in your body responsible for carrying information and clues from your brain and spinal cord out to the rest of your body.

Peripheral neuropathy can be very painful, or you

may experience tingling or numbness in your arms or legs. You may also experience weak muscles or complete or partial loss of control over specific muscles.

Sometimes, peripheral neuropathy can be brought on by a condition other than hypothyroidism.

Research conducted about unexplained neuropathy published in November 2015 in the Muscle & Nerve journal, it was discovered that 0.7 % of peripheral neuropathy were brought on by hypothyroidism versus 25.3% of cases caused by diabetes or prediabetes.

Myxedema

Myxedema is a rare and deadly condition. Undiagnosed hypothyroidism can result in this condition. Signs and symptoms of myxedema include strong cold intolerance and sleepiness followed by significant lethargy and then potential unconsciousness.

A myxedema coma may be brought on by certain sedatives, stress on your body, or infection.

About half of those who develop myxedema will die

from the condition if it is diagnosed too late.

So, if you suspect the situation, seek medical attention as soon as possible.

Carpal Tunnel Syndrome

People with untreated hypothyroidism may also be more prone to carpal tunnel syndrome.

Carpal tunnel syndrome occurs when your median nerve is compressed as it passes into your hand. Your median nerve is the nerve on the palm side of your hand and is often called the carpal tunnel. Your median nerve handles providing feeling to your index finger, long finger, thumb, and a part of your ring finger while it gives off the impulse to your muscle that connects to your thumb.

When your wrist swells, it can cause carpal tunnel syndrome, which will bring on numbness, tingling, or weakness on your hand's side somewhere near your thumb.

https://www.mayoclinic.org/diseases-conditions/hypothyroidism/symptoms-causes/syc-20350284

https://www.everydayhealth.com/hs/hypothyroidis

m/what-happens-if-hypothyroidism-is-left-untreated/

https://www.mayoclinic.org/tests-procedures/thyroidectomy/about/pac-20385195

CHAPTER 7

UNDERSTANDING HYPOTHYROIDISM AND PREGNANCY

It's paramount for all pregnant women with hypothyroidism to have a diagnosis and treatment plan in place. Failure to do so could lead to a myriad of issues.

Pregnancy elicits significant changes in hormones produced by your thyroid gland. As a result, thyroid problems, including hypothyroidism, will usually or sometimes begin with or get worse during pregnancy or after shortly after childbirth.

Hypothyroidism throughout your pregnancy is not prevalent. Hypothyroidism symptoms can sometimes be overlooked because they usually mimic the usual hormonal influences of a typical pregnancy. This includes weight gain and exhaustion.

Alterations in your function can have a negative impact on both the mother and the fetus.

Complications that come to the surface during pregnancy usually depend on the severity of your hypothyroidism. It also depends on how early symptoms were caught, and when the treatment began.

It can also be based on some obstetrical and extragenital pathologies that are linked to the pregnancy.

If the symptoms are caught and treated early enough, it's believed that minimal or no complications will take place during pregnancy.

If the condition is left untreated, maternal hypothyroidism can bring on many risks and complications for both the mother and her baby. We must understand that not only are thyroid hormones' balance imperative for the pregnant woman, but also for the baby's health while it develops.

When hypothyroidism is not treated, pregnant women are susceptible to high blood pressure, low red blood cell count, and severe muscle discomfort and weakness.

There may also be a heightened chance for a miscarried to occur, stillbirth, or premature birth.

Risk Factors

If you are a woman, you are at an increased risk of hypothyroidism if you are over thirty or have prior infertility or preterm delivery, type 1 diabetes, autoimmune disease, or a family history of it.

If you have previous radiation treatment on your neck, head, or past thyroid surgery, you may be at a higher risk. If you have thyroid antibodies such as peroxidase or a goiter, you are also at risk.

If you're currently being treated with levothyroxine, a thyroid hormone drug, it'll need to be adjusted while pregnant.

What are the Causes of Maternal Hypothyroidism?

Hashimoto's disorder is a typical cause of underactive thyroid in pregnant women. Hashimoto's is an autoimmune disease that presents itself when your immune system develops antibodies that work with your immune system. But in this case, those antibodies attack your thyroid. This is what makes your thyroid gland produce an insufficient amount of thyroid hormone.

Other causes of maternal hypothyroidism include being treated for *hyperthyroidism* in the past. This is when the thyroid makes too much thyroid hormone.

In addition, iodine deficiency or having undergone surgery to remove any tumors on your thyroid can lead to maternal hypothyroidism.

Your thyroid also can fail to produce enough thyroid hormone after childbirth. Up to seven percent of women will contract postpartum thyroiditis in her very first year after having her baby. Thyroiditis is known as inflammation of your thyroid gland.

This issue is initiated with hyperthyroidism, which goes away and corrects itself without treatment in a few weeks or months. However, on occasion, the inflammation can go on to be hypothyroidism.

The hypothyroidism will correct itself and go back to normal function on its own. If there's not enough iodine in your diet, it can lead to hypothyroidism. Your thyroid gland relies upon iodine to produce the proper number of thyroid hormones. It should be noted that in the United States, iodine deficiencies are uncommon due to the use of iodized salt. Keep in mind that women who are pregnant or breastfeeding may need more iodine than others and should pay attention to their intake.

How Can Hypothyroidism Affect a Baby in the Womb?

Your baby will rely on you for thyroid hormones during its initial months of your pregnancy.

These hormones from your body are essential for your baby's brain development and growth. As we've noted before that hypothyroidism in the mother may have long-lasting effects on the baby.

How Maternal Hypothyroidism is Treated

The importance of monitoring hypothyroidism throughout pregnancy has been made clear so far.

The most opted treatment for hypothyroidism is a primary thyroid hormone replacement pill with a form of synthetic T4. This synthetic T4, as we know, is called levothyroxine. It's important to note that this medication is the same exact thing and contains the same properties as the T4 your body produces and it's safe for women when they are pregnant.

Before Pregnancy

Thyroid hormone levels must be normal both before and during pregnancy. If you're already taking thyroid medication to treat your thyroid condition, you'll need to to have your thyroid hormone levels analyzed before you try to conceive.

If your TSH levels are too high, you may need an increase in your dose of levothyroxine. You should delay pregnancy until your disease is well controlled.

During Pregnancy

When you have hypothyroidism and get pregnant, your dosage of thyroid medication must be increased because your baby will be taking thyroid hormones from you. Your dosage of the drug may even be increased by up to 30% or more within your initial 4 to 6 weeks of pregnancy. This will be determined by your doctor.

That's why it's important to let your doctor know right away when you do become pregnant.

If you develop hypothyroidism during pregnancy, and this is all brand new to you, you will need your T4 levels to be brought up to a healthy and safe level right away.

Your primary care physician may even provide you with bigger and bigger doses of the medication, levothyroxine until your T4 levels reach a healthy level. After one month after you begin treatment, you must have your thyroid function levels tested again to see where they are.

You should have testing done through your nine months of pregnancy to check your thyroid levels to provide the best pregnancy outcome for you and your baby.

After Pregnancy

After delivering your baby, you can reduce the dosage to average levels again

How to Have a Healthy Baby When You Have Hypothyroidism

Paying attention to both your health and your baby's health can be tough. It's paramount that you work with both your doctor and endocrinologist to develop a treatment plan for the best thyroid monitoring and care *before, during, and after your pregnancy.*

You need to take your thyroid medication as it's

prescribed. Alert your doctor right away about any side effects that you may encounter from the drug.

You must be sure that you are intaking enough iodine. You should be taking daily prenatal vitamins that provide anywhere from 150 to 250 micrograms of potassium iodide or plain iodate.

Please note that if you are breastfeeding, you must take an iodine supplement to ensure that your milk contains enough iodine for your baby.

It is also essential that you don't take your thyroid medication at the same time during the day as you make your prenatal supplements and vitamins that have calcium and iron in them.

Calcium and iron can both interfere with the absorption of your synthetic thyroid hormone. You should take these supplements at least three hours before or after you receive your thyroid medication to be on the safe side.

https://www.healthline.com/health-news/children-thyroid-conditions-raise-pregnancy-risks-052913#1

CHAPTER 8

THE CORRELATION: HYPOTHYROIDISM AND DEPRESSION

So far, we have touched on the link between hypothyroidism and depression a few times. Now, let's go more in-depth and take a look at the correlation between the two.

Some research indicates that there is a direct correlation in people living with hypothyroidism and while also dealing with anxiety and depression. Understanding this link can help create a proper treatment plan that focuses on the physical and mental implications that this condition can cause.

Depression is present in 69 percent of those that have hypothyroidism.

Here's the issue:

Hypothyroidism and depression may display the same symptoms, which could lead the doctors to misdiagnose one for the other.

It can be a vicious cycle to have both since you'll feel very tired, sluggish, and may have trouble focusing and concentrating. As a result, you'll be sleeping a lot more than usual.

Medication

Doctors advise that if you're diagnosed with both, your medication for hypothyroidism will actually help in both cases.

Your thyroid medicine actually boosts the levels of two major thyroid hormones: T3 and T4.

Thyroid Medication and Your Depression

Sometimes your thyroid medication may interfere with any medication that you take for depression. On the flip side, the drug you choose for your depression may be a big player in harming or impacting your thyroid function.

There are many depression or mental health

medications that are known to change your thyroid function.

Hypothyroidism and Your Brain

It's known that your thyroid hormone plays a key and significant role in the development and correct functioning of your brain. T4 is necessary right away for development, but especially during the gestation period for the fetal brain's growth.

Hypothyroidism can also impact or alter your blood flow and how glucose is used in your brain. More so, it is found that those patients who claim to be depressed and display the proper signs of depression can (and sometimes do) have structural aberrations of their hippocampus in their brain. This can bring on defects in the way your memory performs and functions. Moreover, a connection has been found between thyroid peroxidase antibodies (TPO) and depression.

Hypothyroidism and Anxiety

As you already have deduced, hypothyroidism comes with a wide variety of symptoms. Your earliest signs will affect your brain's function as they are psychiatric and usually account for anywhere between 2-12 percent of initial symptoms people encounter when they first become hypothyroid.

These symptoms can include speech issues, trouble staying focused and concentrating, memory lapses, and most notably, anxiety.

In fact, around 40% of those who struggle with hypothyroidism have some form of anxiety disorder.

But it's unknown whether the condition of hypothyroidism actually causes anxiety disorder.

The good news is that it has been documented that individuals with hypothyroidism and anxiety respond very well to treatment with the T4 hormone.

Natural Treatments for Depression and Anxiety

While treating hypothyroidism should help ease symptoms of depression and anxiety, there are some natural ways to quiet the effects of depression and anxiety.

Get Enough Sleep

Depression can either keep you in bed all day, sleep the entire day away, or hinder your sleep.

If this happens and you are missing out on a lot of sleep, you can start trying to correct this by making some simple lifestyle changes.

Try heading to bed and waking up at the same exact time each day. See if you can avoid napping, as this can complicate your sleeping pattern. Remove any computers or televisions from the room you are trying to sleep in to ensure that you do not have any distractions.

Eat Healthy

We know that a healthy lifestyle is a critical player in treating hypothyroidism, but it can also help with depression. Keep in mind that there isn't one specific eating disorder that'll cure depression. Although, we must keep tabs on what you're eating.

If you're one of those, who tend to overeat when upset or depressed, taking control of that pattern can make things better.

As a side note and fun fact, there's evidence that supports that any foods that contain omega-3 fatty acids, such as tuna and salmon, and folic acids, such as avocado and spinach, can assist in helping depression.

Get in a Routine

Finding a routine to slip into can help to reduce feelings of depression. By having a schedule to follow helps to give you structure and purpose.

Set Goals

Start making and setting small goals for yourself, and then move to larger-scale ones.

When you're depressed, you can start to feel worthless, and having and meeting goals can elicit feelings and sensations of accomplishment. Having daily goals for yourself can get you on the right track.

Exercise

Exercise releases those "feel-good" chemicals in your brain that are called endorphins. Training will also deliver some long-term benefits for those who struggle with depression.

Even getting out, walking, and moving around can do a lot of good for your mental health.

Take on Responsibilities

Staying involved in things and having a purpose through the form of daily responsibilities can help to give you a positive outlook and to combat feelings of depression.

Being responsible for things or people can even ground you and give you a warm sense of accomplishment. Feeling important can bring on positive feelings.

Natural Remedies

St. John's Wort

This is a plant that is from Europe, northern Africa, and western Asia. In Europe, St. John's wort is taken to combat depression. But the FDA has not yet approved it for depression.

When you take St. John's wort, you increase the amount of serotonin in your body. Serotonin, like endorphins, is a feel-good chemical in your brain. When people are depressed, they are low in their serotonin levels.

Many types of antidepressants are successful in assisting with depression because they increase the amount of serotonin in your brain.

St. John's wort can sometimes impact other types of medications, such as birth control pills, blood thinners, and chemotherapy medications. So it's advised to always consult with your doctor before supplementing on your own.

Folate

It's believed that having a low level of folic acid in your body is related to depression. Studies have shown that if you supplement with 500 micrograms of folic acid, the effectiveness of depression medication has gone way up. Dark leafy greens, beans, avocados, sunflower seeds, lentils, and fortified cereals are all known to be high in folic acid.

Zinc

Zinc is known to have a correlation with your mental functions like behavior and your learning ability and processing. It's been found that if you are deficient in zinc, it can lead to or worsen depression.

So supplementing with 25 milligrams of zinc daily for about three months can lead to relief from some depression symptoms.

Zinc supplements can also increase your available omega-3 fatty acids in your system.

https://www.webmd.com/depression/features/natural-treatments#1

https://www.healthline.com/health/depression/herbs-supplements#zinc

https://psychopathology.imedpub.com/depression-wellbeing-and-hypothyroidism.php?aid=21181

https://www.medicalnewstoday.com/articles/thyroid-and-depression#summary

CHAPTER 9

HIGH-RISK FACTORS AND WHAT YOU CAN DO ABOUT IT

A risk factor is something that raises your chances of getting a disease or health problem.

You can have or contract hypothyroidism with or without potential risks. Your chances are higher when you have more risk factors.

If you do have some risk factors, you should alert your doctor and work with him or her to devise a plan to reduce them, if possible.

Your family medical history is one of the most common risk factors for hypothyroidism. This is why it's stressed that you need to be knowledgeable about your family history and fill your doctor in.

We also know that significant amounts of iodine in

your diet may also put you at risk for hypothyroidism. Becoming pregnant, being female, or over the age of 60 are also known to be risk factors. Some of the risk factors, like your age and sex, you cannot control or alter. Yet, there are some things you can help by keeping up with your health, exercising, and eating healthy.

Family History

If you have a family history of immune system complications, such as type 1 diabetes, systemic lupus erythematosus, Sjogren syndrome, rheumatoid arthritis, or pernicious anemia, you may be more at risk than others.

While rare, some diseases, such as hemochromatosis, can leave strange substances in your pituitary gland. In the case of hemochromatosis, it's iron that's left behind. This causes central hypothyroidism. Sarcoidosis can cause granuloma deposits in your actual thyroid gland, and this can lead to hypothyroidism as well.

Pamela Allweiss, MD MSPH, an endocrinologist and an assistant professor in family practice at the University of Kentucky College of Medicine in

Lexington states:

*"If you have symptoms related to thyroid disease —
such as depression or anxiety, intolerance to hot or cold
temperatures, or unexpected changes in your weight —
besides the risk factors for thyroid disease, particularly
a family history of autoimmune disease, you should be
screened for thyroid disease."*

*"While not much can be done to prevent thyroid
disease, early detection is important,"* says Dr.
Allweiss. *"Often, thyroid disease symptoms can be
vague, but people with a family history or other thyroid-
disease risk factors should think about [the possibility
of] thyroid disease and talk to their doctor if they notice
any unusual ailments."*

*"If a person has ever been told that they have an
enlarged thyroid or goiter in the past, they should also
be tested for thyroid disease,"* Allweiss states.

*"Prompt diagnosis of thyroid disease is crucial since
there's not much you can do to prevent it, and
treatment is the only way to bring your hormone levels
back into balance."*

What You Need to Know About Thyroid

125

Nodules

Thyroid nodules are bumps and lumps that are forming on your thyroid gland.

Unfortunately, they are ubiquitous. Sometimes, the buds can be cancerous but are usually benign.

Studies and research show that women are way more likely than men to have thyroid nodules.

On the flip side to this, is that men fall susceptible to a much more significant risk to have cancerous nodules.

In any case, a biopsy should always be done.

The risk factors for getting thyroid nodules have hypothyroidism, having Hashimoto's disease, having a diet insufficient in iodine, a family history of thyroid nodules, or a family history of thyroid disease.

Getting checked can assist in finding any thyroid nodules early. If a nodule is found, you may need more testing through a thyroid scan, biopsy, or ultrasound.

Knowing you are at risk for thyroid disease and being upfront and open with your doctor about any signs or symptoms that you pick up on can help for any issues to be found and diagnosed early.

PLEASE LEAVE A REVIEW!

Customer Reviews

⭐⭐⭐⭐⭐ 2
5.0 out of 5 stars ▾

5 star		100%
4 star		0%
3 star		0%
2 star		0%
1 star		0%

See all verified purchase reviews ›

Share your thoughts with other customers

Write a customer review

It would mean so much to me if you could take 60 seconds to leave a brief review on Amazon, even if it's just a few sentences.

I want to make sure this book gets into the hands of as many people as possible to help them.

CONCLUSION

Hypothyroidism is not fun.

It encompasses constant exhaustion, dry skin, possible weight gain, irritability, and mood swings.

If left untreated, these symptoms can impact your mental and physical health as well as your relationships and social life. Your thyroid hormones play a role in about every cell and function of your body. Taking control of your health, whether after years of being diagnosed with hypothyroidism or not, is the first step.

Whatever the case may be, becoming educated is the first step to a healthier lifestyle.

Management is important and with treatment, very manageable.

Your thyroid handles dispersing hormones linked to your energy levels that your body runs off of. When short on energy, you are unable to function. The importance of the thyroid is paramount and you now understand what your body may be going through and the steps to take to begin to feel better.

Feeling better starts with a proper diagnosis, working with both a primary doctor and an endocrinologist who can assist you in setting up a treatment plan. It's important to note that, in aging and in pregnancy, diagnosing the thyroid condition can be tricky and often overlooked or missed because the symptoms that we see in hypothyroidism occur in other illnesses, in aging, and in pregnancy.

You now understand that upon visiting your doctor, you must be in tune with any changes that your body undergoes and to note them so you can present them to your doctor.

Be sure to also provide your doctor with information about any cases of hypothyroidism in your family, your family medical history, previous radiation treatment, your diet, previous thyroid surgeries, and medications that you currently take.

You will need to be examined by your doctor and have bloodwork done to confirm hypothyroidism diagnosis. You now know that this process may involve a lot of trial and error until the proper diagnosis is reached.

Once it's determined that you do have hypothyroidism, you'll need to find the best treatment and dosage of T4, and iodine supplements may or may not be necessary.

Upon diagnosis with hypothyroidism, a change in your diet will most likely be necessary to ensure that you're getting the proper supplementation and being healthy to counteract any unexplained weight gain due to the slow metabolism.

Exercise is also a way to relieve some of the symptoms that come along with the condition.

There are many social and emotional implications and adverse effects of hypothyroidism that can come along with this diagnosis. It has been found that staying active and having a healthy and nutritious diet can help reduce the implications.

Finding relaxation through meditation or yoga is an excellent option for finding a support group or therapist.

You now understand the importance of diet and certain foods to avoid making your symptoms worse or impact your medication's effects. Many foods can help distribute the nutrients necessary to help you better cope with hypothyroidism.

As you should know by now, the goal is to not let your hypothyroidism diagnosis go untreated. As this can bring on many risk factors, including birth defects, goiters, hormone issues, infertility, cardiac problems, and other issues.

It's crucial to recognize that you must stay on top of your thyroid health during pregnancy. When you first become pregnant, the baby will take thyroid hormones from you, and your medication dosage will need to be elevated throughout the pregnancy.

Hypothyroidism is known to affect your mood, and it's not uncommon for those diagnosed with hypothyroidism to struggle with depression.

Your body's thyroid hormone, known as thyroxine (T4), regulates so many aspects of your body that it can lead to significant complications if you don't correct it with T4 supplementation. You realized that there is hope for the future and that living with hypothyroidism can be manageable. Especially if your diagnosis was made early enough before any severe health complications took place.

You have all the information to go forth and take control of your health!

If you found this book to be informative and are

now much more prepared to take on hypothyroidism, please share this with anyone who you know that may suffer from Hypothyroidism.

Another way to provide more exposure for the book would be leaving a review on Amazon.

OTHER BOOKS BY KATHRYN YOUNG

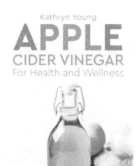

Apple Cider Vinegar For Health and Wellness

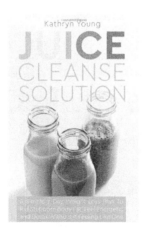

Juice Cleanse Solution

SPECIAL BONUS

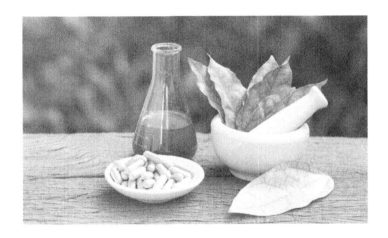

Get the Bonus Report that includes:

❏ Weight loss supplement buying guide
❏ Why **MOST** diets fail
❏ Alternative medicine tricks that worked for me

Get it now, visit the link:

bit.ly/healthybonus

RESOURCES

Chapter 1

American Thyroid Association. 2020. *General Information/Press Room | American Thyroid Association*. Available at: https://www.thyroid.org/media-main/press-room

Yourhormones.info. 2020. *Thyroid Gland | You And Your Hormones From The Society For Endocrinology*. Available at: https://www.yourhormones.info/glands/thyroid-gland/

2020. Health US News. Available at: https://health.usnews.com/health-news/patient-advice/articles/2015/07/21/low-thyroid-in-men-not-just-a-womans-issue

Healthline. 2020. *Autoimmune Diseases: Types, Symptoms, Causes, Diagnosis & More.*
Available at:
https://www.healthline.com/health/autoimmune-disorders#causes

Doheny, K., 2020. *Low Thyroid Level In Newborns: New Clues On How Long To Treat.* [online] EndocrineWeb. Available at:
https://www.endocrineweb.com/conditions/thyroid/low-thyroid-level-newborns-new-clues-how-treat

Publishing, H., 2020. *The Lowdown On Thyroid Slowdown - Harvard Health.* [online] Harvard Health. Available at:
https://www.health.harvard.edu/diseases-and-conditions/the-lowdown-on-thyroid-slowdown

Chapter 2

Thyroid.org. 2020. [online] Available at:
https://www.thyroid.org/wp-content/uploads/patients/brochures/Hypothyroidism_web_booklet.pdf

Publishing, H., 2020. *The Lowdown On Thyroid Slowdown - Harvard Health*. [online] Harvard Health. Available at:
https://www.health.harvard.edu/diseases-and-conditions/the-lowdown-on-thyroid-slowdown

Chapter 3

Welling Homeopathy. 2020. *#1 Doctor For Thyroid Treatment, Homeopathy Medicine For Hypothyroid*. [online] Available at:
https://www.wellinghomeopathy.com/treatment-hypothyroid/#Homeopathic_treatment_forHypothyroid

Healthline. 2020. 5 Natural Remedies For Hypothyroidism. [online] Available at:
https://www.healthline.com/health/hypothyroidism/five-natural-remedies-for-hypothyroidism#gluten-free-diet

Pennstatehershey.adam.com. 2020. *Complementary And Alternative Medicine - Penn State Hershey Medical Center - Hypothyroidism - Penn State Hershey Medical Center*. [online] Available at:

http://pennstatehershey.adam.com/content.aspx?productid=107&pid=33&gid=000093

WebMD. 2020. *Exercises For An Underactive Thyroid*. [online] Available at: https://www.webmd.com/women/features/exercises-underactive-thyroid#1

WebMD. 2020. *How Hypothyroidism Is Treated*. [online] Available at: https://www.webmd.com/women/guide/low-thyroid-treatment#1

Medicalnewstoday.com. 2020. *Hypothyroidism: Causes, Symptoms, And Treatment*. [online] Available at: https://www.medicalnewstoday.com/articles/163729#symptoms

Orenstein, B. and Rosalyn Carson-DeWitt, M., 2020. *Hypothyroidism: When To See An Endocrinologist | Everyday Health*. [online] EverydayHealth.com. Available at: https://www.everydayhealth.com/hs/healthy-living-with-hypothyroidism/see-an-endocrinologist/

Chapter 4

Orenstein, B., & Rosalyn Carson-DeWitt, M. (2020). Getting Support for Hypothyroidism | Everyday Health. Retrieved 23 September 2020, from https://www.everydayhealth.com/hs/healthy-living-with-hypothyroidism/get-support/

Yoga for the Thyroid: 10 Poses to Improve Thyroid Health. (2020). Retrieved 23 September 2020, from https://www.healthline.com/health/yoga-for-thyroid#yoga-poses

Yoga for thyroid problems: 8 poses. (2020). Retrieved 23 September 2020, from https://www.medicalnewstoday.com/articles/320744#beneficial-yoga-poses

Chapter 5

Low thyroid diet strategies that actually work. (2020). Retrieved 23 September 2020, from https://www.precisionnutrition.com/hypothyroidism-diet-plan

What to Eat for Thyroid Health + One Day Thyroid Foods Meal Plan - Dr. Jolene Brighten. (2020). Retrieved 23 September 2020, from https://drbrighten.com/thyroid-foods-and-one-day-thyroid-meal-plan/

Chapter 6

Hypothyroidism - Symptoms and causes. (2020). Retrieved 23 September 2020, from https://www.mayoclinic.org/diseases-conditions/hypothyroidism/symptoms-causes/syc-20350284

Thyroidectomy - Mayo Clinic. (2020). Retrieved 23 September 2020, from https://www.mayoclinic.org/tests-procedures/thyroidectomy/about/pac-20385195

What Happens if Hypothyroidism is Left Untreated? | Everyday Health. (2020). Retrieved 23 September 2020, from https://www.everydayhealth.com/hs/hypothyroidism/what-happens-if-hypothyroidism-is-left-untreated/

Chapter 7

Thyroid Conditions Raise the Risk of Pregnancy Complications. (2020). Retrieved 23 September 2020, from https://www.healthline.com/health-news/children-thyroid-conditions-raise-pregnancy-risks-052913#1

Chapter 8

10 Natural Depression Treatments. (2020). Retrieved 23 September 2020, from https://www.webmd.com/depression/features/natural-treatments#1

6 Herbs and Natural Supplements for Depression. (2020). Retrieved 23 September 2020, from https://www.healthline.com/health/depression/herbs-supplements#zinc

Depression, Well-being and Hypothyroidism. (2020). Retrieved 23 September 2020, from https://psychopathology.imedpub.com/depression-wellbeing-and-hypothyroidism.php?aid=21181

Thyroid and depression: What is the link?. (2020). Retrieved 23 September 2020, from https://www.medicalnewstoday.com/articles/thyroid-and-depression#summary

Made in United States
North Haven, CT
07 May 2024

52219473R00085